Life-Saving Tech

I0477831

Innovations in Early Disease Detection

Emma Royce Smartley

DEDICATION

To the forerunners of medical innovation, whose unwavering quest for information and technology keeps saving lives and influencing healthcare's course.

To the researchers and medical professionals committed to improving early disease detection and giving patients the knowledge and resources they require for improved health.

And may this book help you on your path to a healthy life, to all the people and families that motivate us with their fortitude, optimism, and dedication to wellbeing.

CONTENTS

ACKNOWLEDGMENTS

To everyone who helped create *Life-Saving Tech: Innovations in Early Disease Detection,* I would like to express my sincere gratitude.

I want to start by expressing my gratitude to the medical experts, researchers, and innovators whose innovative work in medical technology served as the inspiration for this book. It is really admirable how dedicated you are to promoting early disease detection and enhancing patient outcomes.

I also want to express my sincere gratitude to my family and friends for their constant encouragement and support along this trip. Your faith in my idea has inspired me to be more creative and determined.

Furthermore, I would like to thank the several writers and academics whose contributions provided the groundwork for the understanding shared here. You have made tremendous contributions to the domains of technology and healthcare.

Finally, thank you to all of the readers who will interact with this work. This effort is motivated by your desire to increase your understanding of early disease detection. I sincerely hope that this book will be a useful tool and encourage you to welcome the advancements that are reshaping the medical field.

CHAPTER 1

THE VALUE OF EARLY HEALTHCARE DETECTION

A key component of efficient healthcare is early detection, which provides the opportunity to cure illnesses before they become life-threatening. Innovative technology and advances in medical science are progressively altering the field of early detection and intervention. This chapter will discuss the many facets of early detection's significance in healthcare, the obstacles that still exist in the early diagnosis of some diseases, and how new technology is propelling advancements in this crucial field.

1.1 Knowing Survival Rates and Early Detection

In the medical field, the idea of early detection is crucial for improving long-term survival and treatment outcomes. Finding an illness early on, before symptoms worsen or spread to other areas of the body, is known as early detection.

Early Detection Definition:

Medical screenings, examinations, and evaluations intended to detect a disease before it reaches an advanced state are referred to as early detection. Early identification can significantly impact treatment options and results for a variety of illnesses, especially cancer. Healthcare professionals can use less invasive therapies with better outcomes and fewer side effects thanks to this proactive approach.

The Effects of Early Detection on Survival Rates:

Early detection greatly increases survival rates for many diseases, including cancer. For instance, when breast cancer is found in its early stages, the five-year survival rate can surpass 90%; but, when the disease is detected later, the percentage drastically decreases. Early action may result in:

- Decreased illness progression helps maintain general health and enjoyment of life.

- The ability of medicines to target smaller, targeted areas results in increased efficacy of treatment.
- Better psychological results for individuals who are aware that their illness is treatable and controllable.

Case Studies on Early vs. Late Detection Survival Rates:

The difference between the results of early and late detection is demonstrated by numerous case studies:

Breast Cancer: Research indicates that the survival rate for breast cancer identified by routine mammography is over 90%, whereas the survival rate for late-stage detection is less than 30%.

The early detection of polyps or malignant growths by routine colonoscopies often enables their removal before they worsen.

The survival rate for prostate cancer that is diagnosed early is about 100%, demonstrating the need of routine examinations.

1.2 Difficulties in Early Disease Detection

Although many illnesses have shown effectiveness with early identification, some diseases still elude early diagnosis because of systemic, biological, and technological obstacles. To advance early detection techniques for a wider range of circumstances, it is imperative to comprehend these obstacles.

Ovarian, lung, and pancreatic cancers that are hard to detect:

Because of their vague or subtle symptoms, some malignancies, including ovarian, lung, and pancreatic tumors, are still challenging to identify in their early stages. For example:

Early identification of pancreatic cancer is difficult since it frequently exhibits no symptoms until it has progressed to an advanced stage.

A persistent cough is one of the moderate signs of lung

cancer that can be confused for other respiratory conditions.

Bloating and stomach pain are examples of ovarian cancer symptoms that are frequently ambiguous, which delays diagnosis.

Delays in diagnosis and technological limitations:

Despite advancements in medical technology, there are still several limitations, especially in imaging and biomarkers:

Sensitivity Issues: Very small tumors or those entrenched in dense tissues may be invisible to imaging technologies.

Limited Biomarkers: There are currently no trustworthy biomarkers that show early onset for some diseases.

Cost and Accessibility: The cost of advanced screening tests can restrict access, particularly in areas with limited resources. Logistical difficulties are further increased by the fact that these examinations frequently call for specific tools and skilled workers.

The Reasons Why Early Detection Is Still Difficult Despite Technological Developments:

Despite advancements in technology, there are a number of reasons why early detection is improving slowly:

Rapid Disease Progression: Some illnesses spread so swiftly that early detection may require more than just routine screening.

Complex Genetic and Environmental Factors: It is challenging to forecast or identify diseases like cancer early using a single method because they can be influenced by a multitude of factors.

Lack of Universal Screening Protocols: Inconsistencies in detection techniques result from the absence of a defined screening protocol for certain conditions.

1.3 The Role of Technology in Early Detection

New opportunities for early disease detection are presented

by emerging healthcare technology. Wearable health technology and artificial intelligence are two examples of developments that are changing the way we approach early detection and assisting in the removal of some of the current obstacles.

Tech-Driven Early Diagnosis Overview:

A variety of diagnostic tools have been made available by technological advancements for faster and more precise detection. Among them are:

Artificial Intelligence (AI): Machine learning algorithms examine patient data and medical imaging to look for early disease indicators, frequently spotting subtleties that human eyes might overlook.

Wearable Health Devices: These gadgets track vital signs and other health indicators, giving constant, real-time information that can reveal illness early warning indications.

Molecular Diagnostics: Methods such as liquid biopsies

examine blood samples for tumor DNA fragments, making it possible to diagnose cancers that would otherwise be difficult to detect.

The Function of Tech Firms and Startups in Healthcare:

Medical institutions are increasingly working with startups and well-established digital companies to develop innovative early detection techniques:

Diagnostic Startups: A lot of startups are concentrating on specialized diagnostics, such as remote monitoring tools that allow for early symptom tracking and wearable biosensors.

Data Analysis Companies: To find possible health hazards, businesses like Google Health and IBM Watson use big data to examine genetic data, imaging, and medical records.

Collaborative Research: To test and validate early detection techniques and expedite development, tech businesses frequently collaborate with hospitals and research institutions.

Technological Solutions Addressing Early Diagnosis:

Cutting-edge technology are being used by creative businesses and research initiatives, with encouraging early detection results:

Mammography AI Systems: AI-powered mammography analysis has demonstrated promise in raising the detection rates of breast cancer, enabling radiologists to identify early warning indications of the disease.

Liquid Biopsy for Cancer: Blood tests that identify cancer-related DNA have been developed by organizations such as Guardant Health, offering a less invasive alternative to conventional biopsies.

Wearable ECG Monitors: FDA-approved ECG technology is now available in devices like the Apple Watch, which may identify irregular heart rhythms that could be signs of early cardiac problems.

A crucial yet complicated aspect of healthcare is early detection, and technology advancements are becoming more and more important in this regard. Even if there are always difficulties, especially with diseases that are difficult to diagnose, the future is bright as long as technology keeps improving. The goal of broad, efficient early detection can be realized with more research, funding, and cooperation, which will ultimately increase survival rates and enhance patients' quality of life everywhere.

CHAPTER 2

DETECTING CANCER USING ARTIFICIAL INTELLIGENCE

By facilitating early diagnosis, individualized therapy, and better results, the use of artificial intelligence (AI) in cancer detection has revolutionized the field of oncology. AI models are increasingly essential for cancer risk assessment and early diagnosis because of their capacity to examine intricate data patterns in sizable medical datasets. This chapter will explore how machine learning is improving cancer imaging, how AI models are transforming cancer prediction, and the potential applications of AI in oncology in the future, along with the ethical issues raised by this development.

2.1 AI-Powered Cancer Prediction Models

AI has demonstrated impressive promise in predicting cancer risk, particularly in those who are more susceptible. Artificial intelligence (AI)-powered models are able to examine complex patterns in medical data and find cancer indications that may be hidden from human view. Cancer prediction has reached new heights thanks to sophisticated AI frameworks like those created at MIT, which show how AI can proactively identify cancer risks.

How AI Models Like Those Developed at MIT Assess Cancer Risk: AI models are being taught to predict cancer risk using genetic, demographic, and lifestyle data at top academic institutes like MIT. These models can identify minor patterns linked to elevated cancer risk by examining past patient data, allowing for the prediction of which people are more likely to develop particular tumors. For example:

- **Breast Cancer Model**s: Artificial intelligence (AI) algorithms have been trained to evaluate patient records and mammography data in order to determine the risk of breast cancer. These algorithms frequently detect possible risks years before any clinical signs manifest.
- AI models evaluate genetic markers, smoking history, and exposure to environmental contaminants to predict lung cancer risk, frequently with a high degree of accuracy.

Training AI on Historical Medical Data: Large datasets from medical records, such as pictures, genetic data, and patient histories, are needed to train AI models for cancer detection. In order to "teach" AI algorithms to identify patterns that might be connected to early-stage malignancies, this data is utilized. The procedure consists of:

- **Data Annotation:** Labeling certain patient data or medical photos to teach AI to distinguish between cancerous and non-cancerous samples.
- Teaching AI to identify patterns in imaging, genetic markers, or symptoms that are associated with increased cancer risk is known as Pattern Recognition.
- **Continuous Learning**: Adding new data to models to keep them accurate and able to adjust to new discoveries.

The Potential of AI for Early Detection in High-Risk Patients: Another important advancement in preventive healthcare is AI's capacity to identify at-risk individuals. High-risk patients, such as those with genetic predispositions or family histories of cancer, can benefit from AI in the following ways:

- **Enable Proactive Surveillance:** Regular screenings based on AI's evaluations can help high-risk individuals catch tumors early.

- **Offer Personalized Health Recommendations:** AI models can further lower the risk of cancer by offering personalized lifestyle advice or preventive steps based on recognized risk factors.

2.2 Cancer Imaging with Machine Learning

Medical imaging in oncology has undergone a revolution thanks to machine learning, especially deep learning. Machine learning algorithms can detect malignant lesions with surprising accuracy by training neural networks on large imaging datasets. This improves diagnosis accuracy and makes early intervention possible.

Deep Learning Applications in Medical Imaging: Deep learning, a branch of machine learning, can identify even the smallest anomalies in medical imaging by using intricate neural networks that replicate human brain activity.

- **Radiology and Pathology:** AI systems examine MRIs, CT scans, X-rays, and pathology slides for signs of cancer, like odd textures or forms that may indicate the existence of tumors.

- **3D Imaging:** AI's capacity to interpret 3D images offers comprehensive information, especially for malignancies in intricate regions like the liver or brain. AI can identify tissue growth or alterations that may point to early cancer stages by comparing photos over time.

Improvements in Cancer Diagnosis Using Machine Learning: By increasing the precision and speed of image interpretation, machine learning models enhance the diagnostic procedure. According to studies, AI-assisted imaging can result in:

- **Increased Diagnostic Accuracy:** AI improves diagnosis accuracy by reducing human error in picture processing, especially for subtle or uncommon cancer forms.

- **Enhanced Detection of Rare malignancies:** Because of their unclear symptoms and body location, some malignancies, such as ovarian or pancreatic, are difficult to detect early. More timely interventions can result from increased early detection rates brought about by machine learning.

- **Decrease in False Positives and Negatives:** Machine learning helps reduce the amount of false positives and negatives, saving patients from needless treatments or delays in critical care.

Case Studies on AI's Predictive Accuracy in Cancer Types: These case studies highlight how AI may be able to identify cancer more accurately than conventional diagnostic techniques.

- **Breast Cancer diagnosis**: A recent study showed that an AI model improved the accuracy of early diagnosis for breast cancer by reducing false-positive rates in mammography by over 10%.

- The application of AI models in lung CT scans has enhanced the identification of tiny nodules that human radiologists might miss, allowing for the early diagnosis of lung cancer.

- **Melanoma Identification:** Machine learning models trained on skin pictures have identified melanoma, a lethal skin cancer, with over 90% accuracy, frequently more accurately than dermatologists.

2.3 AI's Potential in Oncology in the Future

Further developments in precision medicine, early-stage cancer detection, and individualized treatment regimens are anticipated as AI in oncology advances. But as these technologies develop, it becomes more crucial than ever to address the moral and legal issues pertaining to AI's use in healthcare.

AI Advances for Precision Oncology: Precision oncology is a patient-centered approach that customizes therapy regimens according to each patient's unique genetic, environmental, and lifestyle characteristics. AI helps with this by:

- **Genomic Data Analysis**: AI-powered systems examine genomic data to identify genetic alterations connected to particular cancer kinds, enabling more specialized therapies.
- Predictive modeling for treatment outcomes allows

doctors to customize treatment plans and reduce side effects by using AI models to forecast how various patients may react to particular treatments.

- AI can speed up the creation of new cancer medications or find novel applications for already-approved medications, improving therapy options for patients with uncommon or resistant tumors.

Expanding AI Applications to Various Cancer Types: Although AI has shown promise in identifying common diseases such as lung and breast cancer, its uses are growing to include more difficult and uncommon cancer types:

- **Blood malignancies:** AI models are being trained to examine molecular markers and blood tests in order to identify blood malignancies, including lymphoma and leukemia, even when they are asymptomatic.

- **Neurological Tumors:** Since tiny abnormalities might be challenging to detect manually, AI is being used more and more to diagnose brain tumors.

- **Gastrointestinal tumors:** In order to identify tumors in the digestive tract, where early diagnosis has historically been difficult, researchers are using AI in endoscopic and imaging applications.

Ethical Considerations in AI-Driven Healthcare: A number of ethical concerns surface as AI is increasingly incorporated into cancer diagnosis and treatment:

- **Data Privacy and Consent:** Strict privacy rules must be followed while handling patient data in order to protect patient rights, even though it is essential for training AI models. AI creators and medical professionals need to make sure that informed consent is acquired and that data usage is transparent.

- AI models are only as objective as the data they are educated on, which is known as algorithmic bias. If certain demographic biases are reflected in historical data, the AI may unintentionally generate biased conclusions. In order to guarantee equitable healthcare, these biases must be addressed.

- **Human Oversight:** Although AI can provide exceptional diagnostic support, human knowledge should always be complemented, not replaced. Maintaining clinical judgment and responsibility requires involving healthcare practitioners in AI-driven choices.

- **Cost and Accessibility:** Advanced AI tools can be costly, which raises questions about fair access to AI-driven treatment, particularly for marginalized groups. In order to prevent the healthcare disparities gap from growing, efforts should be made to democratize AI technologies.

From precision oncology for individualized treatment to predictive models for early detection, AI's role in cancer detection has revolutionary potential. AI will probably reshape oncology procedures, enhance patient outcomes, and enable more efficient and individualized cancer therapy as it develops. But these developments also bring with them ethical obligations that legislators, healthcare professionals, and AI developers must meet to guarantee that the advantages of AI are equitable, available, and applied in ways that put patient welfare first.

CHAPTER 3

EARLY DIAGNOSIS USING NANOTECHNOLOGY

Innovative developments in medical diagnostics are being propelled by nanotechnology, a discipline that works with matter at the atomic and molecular level. It has amazing promise for early illness detection, frequently with sensitivity and accuracy that are not possible with conventional techniques. This chapter examines the use of nanotechnology in illness detection, the introduction of smartphone-enabled phase imaging, and the technology's potential for easily accessible, non-invasive at-home testing in the future.

3.1 Using Nanotechnology to Identify Diseases

Early diagnosis and better patient outcomes are now possible because of the development of highly sensitive and specific disease detection techniques made possible by nanotechnology. Working at the nanoscale allows researchers to create instruments and materials that directly interact with biological molecules, identifying anomalies that indicate the existence of illnesses even at the subcellular level.

Basic Principles of Nanotechnology in Diagnostics: Nanotechnology manipulates materials that are roughly a thousand times smaller than a cell, operating on a scale of 1 to 100 nanometers. Materials' characteristics drastically alter at this level, enabling special interactions with biological molecules.

- **Enhanced Sensitivity:** Even at extremely low concentrations, nanoparticles can be engineered to bind selectively to certain biomarkers, which are chemicals that indicate the existence of a disease.

- **Targeted Interactions:** By highlighting sick tissues or infections, functionalized nanoparticles which are made with chemicals that target particular cells or proteins can improve diagnostic accuracy.

Important Uses of Nanotechnology in Healthcare: Nanotechnology is being used in a variety of diagnostic fields, including infectious illnesses and oncology.

- **Cancer Detection:** Biomarkers linked to different types of cancer are being found using nanoparticles. For example, gold nanoparticles have the ability to adhere to cancer cells and increase their visibility during imaging, which helps in early diagnosis.

- **Infectious Disease Screening:** Diagnostic instruments based on nanotechnology can identify bacteria and viruses early in the course of an infection. For instance, COVID-19 proteins can be quickly and sensitively detected using nanoparticle assays.

- **Neurological Disease Markers:** In order to diagnose neurological disorders like Alzheimer's disease before clinical symptoms appear, nanoparticles are also being investigated for their ability to identify biomarkers.

Miniaturizing Diagnostic Tools with Nanotechnology: Nanotechnology makes it possible to reduce the size of diagnostic instruments, producing portable, user-friendly instruments that may be used outside of hospital environments.

- **Point-of-Care Devices:** Nanotechnology makes it

possible to create small, portable instruments for quick diagnosis. These instruments are perfect for emergency situations or isolated locations with limited access to healthcare facilities.

- **Lab-on-a-Chip Technologies:** These gadgets combine multiple laboratory operations onto a single microchip, allowing them to examine tiny blood or saliva samples for signs of illness. Lab-on-a-chip technologies provide real-time results, lower expenses, and increase accessibility.

3.2 Phase Imaging Assisted by Smartphones

A new technology called smartphone-enabled phase imaging incorporates phase imaging features into commonplace gadgets like cell phones. Phase imaging is a potential technique for quick and easy diagnostics since it enables the fine-grained viewing of cells and tissues without the need for dyes or labels.

How Phase Imaging Works: The idea behind phase imaging is to identify changes in light as it travels through various things, such tissues or cells. Because biological materials frequently differ in density, light refracts differently through them.

- **Label-Free Imaging:** Phase imaging preserves biological samples in their natural condition and is perfect for sensitive cell examination because it doesn't require dyes or stains like standard microscopy does.

- The ability of phase imaging to discern subtle variations in cell structure is crucial for spotting early cellular alterations linked to illness.

Adapting Phase Imaging for Smartphone Use: Phase imaging technology has been modified for smartphones thanks to recent developments, allowing for quick and easy diagnostics on widely accessible devices.

- **Integrated Microscope Attachments:** Users can take detailed pictures of cells and tissues with the use of miniature microscope attachments for smartphones that can conduct high-resolution phase imaging.

- **AI-Enhanced Image Analysis:** Smartphone-based phase imaging, when combined with AI algorithms, can analyze images to identify anomalies and categorize illness signs, bringing advanced diagnostics to the general public.

- **User-Friendly Interface:** Apps for smartphone-enabled phase imaging make the procedure easier for users by providing clear results and recommendations for next steps in the event that anomalies are found.

Implications for Accessible At-Home Diagnostics: Phase imaging enabled by smartphones makes at-home diagnostics more economical and accessible.

- **Wider Reach:** This technology democratizes access to diagnostic instruments, enabling those in under-resourced or rural places to get high-quality healthcare.
- **Early Intervention:** People who have access to phase imaging can keep a closer eye on their health and treat illnesses sooner rather than later.

3.3 Nanotechnology's Prospects for At-Home Testing

Nanotechnology's role in diagnostics is developing quickly, with an emphasis on non-invasive, at-home testing methods that can screen for a variety of illnesses. With the goal of enabling people to take charge of their health in real time, this development signifies a paradigm shift in the healthcare industry.

Advances in Nanotechnology for Non-intrusive Testing: By doing away with the need for needles, biopsies, or other invasive procedures, non-invasive testing reduces discomfort and increases patient compliance.

- **Breath Analysis:** Nanotechnology tools are being created to examine breath for biomarkers linked to diseases such as liver disease, lung cancer, and even metabolic disorders. These gadgets identify trace gasses linked to particular illnesses by using sensors covered with nanoparticles.

- The creation of portable devices that can examine saliva or urine for early illness signs, such as some infections and malignancies, is made possible by nanotechnology. This makes diagnostics as easy as supplying a little sample at home.

Potential Diseases Detectable with Nanotechnology: Nanotechnology's adaptability enables it to target a variety of illnesses, such as:

- **Cancer:** Early identification of cancers such as pancreatic, breast, and prostate cancers is made possible by nanoparticles' ability to identify tumor markers in physiological fluids.

- **Cardiovascular Diseases:** Nanotech instruments are being created to identify biomarkers, including proteins released after arterial injury, that are connected to heart disease.

- **Diabetes and Metabolic Disorders:** Non-invasive blood glucose monitoring is possible with nanoparticle sensors, offering a less complicated option for managing diabetes.

- **Infectious Diseases:** Nanotechnology has demonstrated potential in quickly identifying microorganisms linked to illnesses like influenza, TB, and HIV, allowing people to get prompt feedback and take the appropriate precautions.

Challenges and Regulatory Hurdles: Although nanotechnology has a lot of potential, a number of issues and regulations need to be resolved before these solutions are widely adopted.

- The safety and biocompatibility of nanoparticles used in diagnostics are crucial because some of them may build up in tissues or interact with biological systems in unpredictable ways.

- **Standardization of Nanotech Devices:** To guarantee accuracy and dependability across various devices and brands, standardization of nanotech diagnostic devices is essential. Guidelines must be set by regulatory agencies to ensure that these gadgets operate reliably.

- **Privacy and Data Security:** Data privacy is a major problem when using at-home diagnostic gadgets that are connected to cell phones or cloud-based services. Sensitive health information must be protected by regulatory frameworks that make sure it is kept safe and distributed only to those who are permitted.

- The early development costs of nanotech-based diagnostics are substantial, despite the fact that they have the potential to save healthcare costs. Prioritizing pricing and accessibility is still an issue for industry stakeholders, especially in low-income areas.

Nanotechnology promises early, non-invasive disease diagnosis that may be done from the comfort of one's home, marking a revolutionary advancement in medical diagnostics. This technology has the potential to improve healthcare by becoming more proactive, accessible, and customized as it advances. Although there are still obstacles to overcome, particularly in the areas of safety and regulation, the use of nanotechnology in diagnostics appears to have a bright future. By enabling the early detection and treatment of illnesses, it might have a substantial impact on public health.

CHAPTER 4

AT-HOME TESTING USING SMARTPHONE TECHNOLOGY

By changing how patients manage and track their health, smartphone technology has completely changed the healthcare sector. Smartphone-enabled at-home diagnostic tools, in particular, provide previously unheard-of access to health information and enable people to take charge of their health. The development of at-home diagnostic tools is examined in this chapter, along with a case study of Healthy.io's Minuteful Kidney Test. It also looks at the wider prospects for smartphone diagnostics in the healthcare industry.

4.1 The Development of Home Diagnostic Instruments

Recent years have seen a substantial evolution in at-home diagnostic instruments, with more precise, practical, and affordable testing alternatives made possible by advances in mobile technology. There are many advantages to the move to smartphone-enabled diagnostics, including patient empowerment and proactive healthcare.

Growth of At-Home Health Testing: Previously, only simple tools like blood pressure monitors and thermometers could be used for at-home health testing. These days, patients can perform more tests at home thanks to smartphone technology, which enables real-time disease screening and chronic condition monitoring.

- **Historical Context:** Simple point-of-care devices, including glucometers for diabetes treatment, were the first to introduce the idea of at-home diagnostics. However, at-home testing possibilities have been greatly increased by the widespread use of smartphones, the development of advanced sensors, and AI-driven algorithms.

- **Technological Enablers**: Using a smartphone to do complex diagnostic tests is now feasible because of developments in mobile sensors, artificial intelligence, and cloud computing. Real-time data analysis is made possible by these technologies, which also link patients to medical experts and offer useful insights.

Benefits of Smartphone-Based Diagnostics: As diagnostic instruments, smartphones provide a number of advantages that improve patient satisfaction and healthcare quality.

- **Convenience and Accessibility:** Patients can do tests from the comfort of their homes with smartphone diagnostics, which eliminates the need for frequent clinic visits and increases accessibility for people living in rural or underserved areas.

- **Cost-Effectiveness:** By eliminating the need for in-person consultations, laboratory services, and travel fees, at-home testing can drastically reduce healthcare costs.

- **Real-Time Data gathering:** Smartphone-based diagnostics enable real-time data gathering, which over time offers a more complete picture of a patient's health. This makes it possible to provide individualized treatment and identify possible health problems early.

Patient Empowerment Through Smartphone Tech: The empowerment that smartphone diagnostics offers patients is among its most revolutionary features.

- The transition from reactive to proactive healthcare is made possible by smartphone-based diagnostics, which enable patients to monitor their health metrics more frequently and spot problems before they get out of hand.

- **More Health Literacy:** Smartphone apps that provide clear, concise results and guided instructions enhance health literacy, assisting patients in making well-informed healthcare decisions.

- **Enhanced Doctor-Patient Communication**: Smartphone diagnostics let patients and doctors have educated conversations, which results in more individualized and efficient treatment regimens, by producing data that can be shared directly with healthcare professionals.

4.2 Case Study: Healthy.io's Minuteful Kidney Test

A cutting-edge example of smartphone-enabled diagnostic equipment that enables patients to keep an eye on their kidney health from home is Healthy.io's Minuteful Kidney Test. The test serves as an example of how AI and computer vision are used to produce dependable, accurate results in an approachable manner.

The Minuteful Kidney Test is a straightforward urine test that can be performed at home using a smartphone camera and a related software to check for kidney disease symptoms.

- The patient must gather a urine sample and dip a test strip into it in order to perform the test. The smartphone's camera is then used to scan the strip once it has been placed on a color-coded board.

- **Smartphone Camera and Color Analysis:** The app takes a picture of the test strip using the camera on the smartphone and analyzes color changes on the strip to determine whether certain biomarkers linked to kidney disease are present.

- **Ease of Use:** Even individuals with little technical expertise may use the app because it has an intuitive UI and step-by-step instructions.

AI and Computer Vision in Analyzing Test Results: By examining color variations on the test strip, the Minuteful Kidney Test uses AI and computer vision to provide precise results.

- **Advanced Algorithms:** To ensure accurate readings, the app employs computer vision algorithms to interpret the colors on the test strip, accounting for angle and lighting.
- The use of machine learning models reduces the possibility of false positives or negatives by improving reading accuracy and consistency through the use of AI algorithms trained on thousands of test samples.
- **Automated Reporting:** After the analysis is finished, the app creates a report that is simple to share with medical professionals, enabling timely follow-up care if necessary.

Patient Experiences and Outcomes: Patients, especially those at risk for chronic kidney disease, have shown encouraging results with the Minuteful Kidney Test.

- **Increased Screening Rates:** Patients who might have otherwise postponed testing can now receive early intervention for kidney disease thanks to the accessibility of at-home testing.
- **Improved Patient Compliance:** Patients are more

willing to perform tests at home rather than attend the clinic on a frequent basis, which results in improved chronic kidney condition monitoring and management.

- The test's accuracy, convenience, and ease of use are highlighted in user feedback, and many patients express gratitude for the chance to independently monitor their health.

4.3 Future Health Applications and Smartphone Diagnostics

Smartphone diagnostics has the potential to grow in many healthcare domains in the future, offering more comprehensive testing choices and guaranteeing proactive and accessible healthcare.

It is anticipated that the range of at-home testing will increase as smartphone diagnostics make it possible to conduct more intricate and varied tests.

- **Blood and Biomarker Analysis:** Thanks to developments in smartphone technology, it may soon be possible to perform blood tests and biomarker analyses at home to identify metabolic disorders, anemia, and abnormalities in liver function.

- **Infectious Disease Screening:** At-home screening for infectious diseases, such as COVID-19, influenza, and STIs, may be made possible by smartphone diagnostics, which would speed up diagnosis and lessen the transmission of these illnesses across the community.

- **Genetic and Molecular Testing**: New advancements could integrate genetic and molecular diagnostics into smartphone-based systems, enabling people to check for molecular markers linked to certain diseases and genetic predispositions.

Scaling Smartphone Diagnostics Across Healthcare: Collaborations between tech firms, healthcare providers, and regulatory agencies are necessary to scale smartphone diagnostics throughout the healthcare system.

- In order to provide smooth care coordination, healthcare providers can obtain patients' diagnostic data in real time by integrating smartphone diagnostics with electronic health records (EHRs).

- **Telemedicine Compatibility**: As telemedicine

grows, smartphone diagnostics offer helpful assistance by enabling patients to conduct tests from a distance and exchange information with their doctors during online consultations.

- **Collaborations with Health Systems:** By working together, technology firms and healthcare providers may hasten the uptake of smartphone diagnostics, facilitating widespread implementation and guaranteeing that the technology reaches a wide range of patients.

Addressing Privacy and Accuracy in Smartphone Diagnostics: As smartphone diagnostics proliferate, it will be critical to protect data privacy and preserve diagnostic precision.

- **Data Privacy and Security:** To preserve patient privacy and comply with laws such as the General Data Protection Regulation (GDPR) and the Health Insurance Portability and Accountability Act (HIPAA), personal health data must be safeguarded.

- **Accuracy and Reliability Standards:** To prevent misdiagnosis and guarantee patient safety, smartphone diagnostic accuracy must be guaranteed.

Businesses creating these technologies have to follow strict legal requirements and go through a rigorous clinical validation process.

- To enable customers to make educated decisions regarding their privacy and healthcare, it is imperative that businesses are open and honest about the ways in which they gather, keep, and utilize patient data.

At-home testing has been reimagined by smartphone technology, giving patients more control over their health and better access to diagnostic resources. Smartphone diagnostics can be used for a wide range of purposes, from genetic testing to chronic disease monitoring, thanks to developments in AI, machine learning, and mobile technology. Focusing on data privacy, accuracy, and accessibility will be essential as the healthcare sector adopts these advances in order to foster trust and guarantee the long-term viability of smartphone diagnostics. A future where healthcare is accessible, convenient, and tailored at the push of a button is promised by the advancement of smartphone technology.

CHAPTER 5

TECHNOLOGIES FOR BIOMARKER-BASED DETECTION

Through the identification of biological markers linked to certain medical disorders, biomarker-based detection technologies have completely changed early diagnosis and illness management. These technologies improve the accuracy and speed of illness detection by enabling highly tailored and focused diagnostics. The function of biomarkers in diagnostics, the development of lab-on-a-chip technology, and the funding environment that is propelling the expansion of biomarker-based early detection are all covered in this chapter.

5.1 Biomarkers' Function in the Identification of Disease

Biomarkers are quantifiable markers of biological states or processes that aid in the diagnosis of diseases at different stages, prognostication of patient outcomes, and direction of therapy regimens. Biomarkers have drawn attention recently as potent diagnostic tools that enable more precise and individualized healthcare strategies.

Introduction to Biomarkers in Diagnostics: Biomarkers can be anything from complicated biological patterns that can be detected by imaging to particular molecules present in tissue, blood, or saliva. These signs are perfect for early diagnosis and monitoring because they are frequently present at various phases of the disease progression.

- **Definition and Significance** Biomarkers are quantifiable biological characteristics that can reveal whether a physiological process is normal or pathological. Proteins, DNA, and other substances that indicate the existence or probability of a disease are among them.

- **Clinical Utility:** Because biomarkers may confirm a diagnosis, forecast disease risk, and even anticipate a patient's potential response to a particular treatment, they are essential to the shift toward precision medicine.

Types of Biomarkers for Different Diseases: Biomarkers

differ based on the disease and its distinct biological footprint; they are not universal. Knowing the many kinds of biomarkers makes it easier to customize diagnostics for particular ailments.

1. **Genomic Biomarkers:** These are genetic markers that can show amplifications, deletions, or mutations linked to genetic illnesses or diseases like cancer.

2. Proteomic biomarkers, which are unique proteins or patterns present in physiological fluids, are frequently used to identify neurological disorders, cardiovascular ailments, and malignancies.

3. **Metabolic Biomarkers:** These indicators provide insight into the body's metabolic activities and aid in the diagnosis of conditions linked to obesity, diabetes, and liver disease.

These signs, known as immunological biomarkers, quantify immune responses and aid in the identification of infections, autoimmune illnesses, and even the tracking of organ transplant rejection.

Biomarker-Based Diagnostics Benefits: Biomarker-based diagnostics are a popular option for early illness detection and management due to its many advantages over conventional diagnostic techniques.

- Better patient outcomes and higher survival rates can result from the use of biomarkers to identify diseases in their earliest stages, even before symptoms manifest.

- **Non-Invasive Testing:** Compared to tissue biopsies or surgical procedures, many biomarker tests are less invasive since they use samples of blood, urine, or saliva.

- **Personalized Medicine:** By identifying how a person's particular biology will react to particular treatments, biomarkers assist in customizing care for each patient.

- **Decreased Healthcare Costs:** By facilitating prompt action, early and precise diagnostics can lessen the need for expensive surgeries and drawn-out therapies.

5.2 Technology on a Chip

By condensing laboratory operations onto a single microchip, lab-on-a-chip (LOC) technology enables the rapid, precise, and frequently less expensive execution of complex diagnostic tests. By developing portable and effective testing systems, particularly for cancer and other severe illnesses, this technology has revolutionized biomarker testing.

Overview of Lab-on-a-Chip Systems: Lab-on-a-chip technology is perfect for point-of-care diagnostics because it combines biosensing and microfluidics techniques to reproduce whole lab workflows on a small device.

- **Microfluidics-Based Diagnostics:** LOC devices can manipulate small volumes of fluid (such as blood or saliva) by using microfluidics, which simplifies sample preparation, mixing, and analysis on a single platform.

- **Benefits of LOC in Healthcare:** Compared to conventional laboratory setups, lab-on-a-chip devices are faster, smaller, and use less reagents. They are appropriate for population-wide screening programs since they can also be used for high-throughput screening.

- **Applications Across Disease Types**: LOC technology is very flexible and can be set up for a range of biomarker-based tests, including those for cancer, chronic illnesses, and infectious diseases.

How Biological Dynamics' Pancreatic Cancer Test Operates: Biological Dynamics has created a novel lab-on-a-chip test for pancreatic cancer, a condition that is infamously hard to identify in its early stages. The ability of lab-on-a-chip technology to target particular biomarkers for fatal malignancies is demonstrated by this LOC test.

- The test isolates extracellular vesicles (EVs) from a blood sample in order to perform the detection mechanism. The disease-specific biomarkers carried by these EVs are subsequently examined for indications of pancreatic cancer.

- **Technological Integration**: The test offers a non-invasive and effective diagnostic alternative by rapidly identifying EVs linked to pancreatic cancer by fusing microfluidics and machine learning.

- **Impact on Patient Outcomes:** Since pancreatic cancer frequently goes undetected until it is advanced, early identification is essential to increasing survival rates. A better prognosis and earlier action are made possible by Biological Dynamics' LOC test, which can identify the illness in its early stages.

Scaling Lab-on-a-Chip for Various malignancies: Due to the versatility of lab-on-a-chip technology, it is possible to create comparable tests for additional malignancies that target particular biomarkers linked to various tumor types.

- **Prostate Cancer**: Prostate-specific antigen (PSA) levels in blood can be detected using LOC technology, which offers a quicker and easier substitute for conventional lab-based PSA testing.

- **Breast Cancer:** Personalized breast cancer diagnoses are provided by LOC devices that identify hormone receptor biomarkers, including HER2 and estrogen receptors, which help inform therapy choices.

- **Lung Cancer**: LOC technology is being used to study biomarkers such circulating tumor cells (CTCs), which may allow for less invasive lung cancer identification.

5.3 Biomarker Technology Funding and Development

Both public and private sector investment and innovation

are critical to the development of biomarker-based detection technology. Investments have increased as a result of growing knowledge of biomarker efficacy in diagnostics, which is driving research and development to improve and broaden the use of biomarkers in a variety of diseases.

Investment Trends in Biomarker Technology: Big pharmaceutical corporations, government funding, and venture capital have all made major investments in biomarker-based diagnostics. This funding is essential for expanding research and developing cutting-edge technology.

- **Government Grants and Initiatives:** As part of public health campaigns to save healthcare costs through preventative medicine, governments around the world are funding biomarker research. The National Institutes of Health (NIH), for instance, provides funding for studies on biomarkers related to cardiovascular and cancer conditions.

- In order to create companion diagnostics tests that help ascertain whether patients are likely to respond to a specific medication many pharmaceutical companies engage in biomarker technology. Better patient outcomes and more focused treatment are made possible by this.

- **Venture Capital and Startups:** Because biomarker technology has the potential to revolutionize healthcare, venture capitalists are increasingly funding biomarker startups. Because of the market's need for early detection solutions and their potential impact on precision medicine, biomarker firms frequently secure investment.

Success Stories and Promising Startups: A number of established businesses and startups have made noteworthy advances in biomarker technology, providing fresh methods for illness monitoring and detection.

- **Grail:** A business that specializes in early cancer diagnosis, Grail's multi-cancer screening test looks for genetic changes linked to several cancer types using a blood sample.
- With an emphasis on colorectal cancer screening, the startup Freenome uses biomarker technology and machine learning to detect early-stage tumors from blood testing.

- **Caris Life Sciences:** With a focus on thorough molecular profiling, Caris advances individualized cancer care by using biomarker data to inform cancer therapy choices.

- **Nanostring Technologies:** Distinguished by its emphasis on gene expression profiling, Nanostring creates diagnostic tests that identify diseases, such as autoimmune disorders and cancer, using genetic biomarkers.

The Future of Biomarker-Based Early Detection: Research is being conducted to increase the capabilities of biomarkers and make diagnostics even more accurate, available, and economical. This bodes well for the future of biomarker-based detection technologies.

- The development of panels that examine many biomarkers at the same time may provide thorough health screening in a single test, increasing patient compliance and detection rates.

- **AI Integration:** In order to analyze complicated biomarker data, find trends that traditional analysis techniques might overlook, and eventually increase diagnostic accuracy, artificial intelligence will be essential.

- **Global Accessibility and Affordability:** Efforts are underway to lower the costs of these tests as biomarker technology develops. This will be essential for democratizing access to early detection by introducing biomarker-based testing to underserved areas and lower-income groups.

- **Regulatory Advancements:** To safely introduce novel tests to the market, the quick speed of biomarker discovery necessitates a flexible regulatory environment. The FDA and other regulatory bodies are creating recommendations to expedite the biomarker approval process while maintaining accuracy and dependability.

Biomarker-based detection technologies are opening the door to healthcare that is more individualized, accurate, and easily accessible. From lab-on-a-chip advancements that facilitate quick cancer detection to the strong funding environment supporting research into next-generation technologies, the use of biomarkers in diagnostics has revolutionary potential. By detecting diseases earlier and more precisely, biomarker-based diagnostics have the potential to revolutionize early detection and intervention, improving outcomes and saving lives.

CHAPTER 6

AI in the Identification of Non-Cancer Diseases

By improving disease diagnosis, treatment planning, and prognosis, artificial intelligence (AI) has completely changed the healthcare industry. Although AI is frequently linked to oncology, its uses in the diagnosis of non-cancerous diseases are just as revolutionary. This chapter explores the expanding use of AI in the diagnosis of infectious, neurological, cardiovascular, and mental health conditions. AI makes it possible for earlier identification, customized treatment, and real-time monitoring to better control these pervasive health conditions by utilizing enormous databases and prediction algorithms.

6.1 AI in the Prediction of Cardiovascular Disease

Since cardiovascular disease (CVD) is still one of the world's leading causes of mortality, new strategies for early detection and prevention are required. By detecting high-risk individuals, evaluating enormous volumes of patient data, and creating individualized therapy suggestions, artificial intelligence has become a vital tool in cardiovascular health.

AI Applications in Predicting Heart Disease: AI-driven models find patterns linked to cardiovascular disease risk factors by analyzing massive datasets, such as imaging, laboratory testing, and electronic health records (EHRs). These models are remarkably accurate at predicting the risk of heart attacks, strokes, and other cardiovascular events.

- EHRs, genetic data, and imaging results are just a few examples of the types of data that AI algorithms, especially deep learning models, can examine to find intricate patterns that predict the risk of CVD.
- AI is able to investigate a greater range of indications, including non-traditional markers like stress levels, physical activity patterns, and social determinants of health. Traditional risk assessments concentrate on specific criteria (e.g., age, cholesterol levels).

- **prediction Models:** By continuously learning from fresh data, machine learning models particularly neural networks can attain high prediction accuracy. By analyzing hundreds of factors at once, these models are able to identify links that human specialists frequently overlook.

Early Detection for High-Risk Cardiovascular Conditions: Proactive management of cardiovascular risks is made possible by early detection, which lowers death rates and stops the course of disease.

- **Hypertension and Atherosclerosis Detection:** By examining minute variations in blood pressure, cholesterol, and other physiological markers over time, AI can detect people who are at risk for diseases like hypertension or atherosclerosis.

- **ECG and Imaging Analysis**: To identify early indicators of heart illness, artificial intelligence (AI) systems can evaluate electrocardiograms (ECG) and imaging data, including CT and MRI scans. An AI system may, for instance, identify early plaque accumulation or abnormal heart rhythms that could result in serious cardiovascular catastrophes.

- **Wearable Technology Integration:** Wearables with AI capabilities, such as smartwatches, can track blood pressure, oxygen levels, and heart rate in real time, warning users of possible cardiac events and facilitating prompt medical intervention.

Case Studies and Patient Outcomes: Several case studies show how AI has improved cardiovascular care, resulting in lower hospitalization rates and better patient outcomes.

- In order to identify asymptomatic left ventricular dysfunction, a sign of heart failure, the Mayo Clinic created an AI-driven program that utilizes ECG data. By facilitating early intervention, this technology has assisted patients in halting the advancement of cardiac disease.

- **Google's Heart Disease Prediction algorithm:** This effective and non-invasive screening technology has demonstrated high accuracy in clinical trials thanks to Google's deep learning algorithm, which uses retinal pictures to predict heart disease risk.

- **Patient Impact:** As people become more aware of their cardiovascular health and the hazards they face, these AI applications have improved patient adherence to treatment regimens.

6.2 AI in Mental and Neurological Conditions

In areas where conventional diagnostic techniques frequently fail to identify complicated neurological and mental health disorders, artificial intelligence has demonstrated potential. AI advances customized mental healthcare by enabling early identification of neurodegenerative illnesses and providing predictive models for mental health issues through the analysis of imaging data, genetic markers, and patient behavior.

Identifying Early Indications of Alzheimer's and Other Neurological Disorders: Neurodegenerative illnesses such as Parkinson's and Alzheimer's are frequently hard to identify in their early stages, which causes treatment to be postponed. By analyzing symptoms and identifying patterns in imaging data, AI opens the door to early detection.

- **Imaging-Based Detection:** Artificial intelligence systems examine brain scans, such as MRIs and PET scans, to find patterns that point to neurodegeneration, frequently years before symptoms manifest. Early atrophy in particular brain regions, for example, may indicate a higher chance of Alzheimer's disease.

- **Behavioral and Cognitive Analysis:** AI can identify early indicators of neurological degeneration by tracking minute alterations in a patient's speech, movement, and cognitive capacities. For instance, non-invasive techniques like voice and gait analysis are becoming popular for identifying those who are at risk.

- **Genomic Insights:** AI can detect people who are at risk of neurodegenerative illnesses by examining genetic markers, allowing for individualized preventative care.

AI-Based Predictive Models for Mental Health: Accurately diagnosing mental health problems, such as schizophrenia, anxiety, and depression, can be difficult. Predictive models powered by AI provide new instruments for early detection and intervention.

- **Natural Language Processing (NLP):** NLP

algorithms can recognize symptoms of depression, anxiety, or suicidal thoughts by analyzing a patient's speech patterns, vocabulary, and tone in written notes, social media posts, and therapy sessions.

- **Behavioral Monitoring:** Wearable AI technology can monitor behavioral indicators including social engagement, physical activity, and sleep patterns, enabling doctors to make real-time assessments of a patient's mental health.

- **Machine Learning for Diagnosis and Prediction:** To assist doctors in proactive treatment and intervention planning, machine learning models evaluate intricate data from patient histories and behavioral patterns to forecast the possibility of mental health disorders.

Integrating AI for Early Diagnosis and Personalized Treatment: By evaluating patient-specific data, AI helps physicians create individualized treatment plans, offering a more focused approach to neurological and mental health care.

- **Personalized Cognitive Behavioral Therapy (CBT):** AI systems can suggest tailored CBT methods according to the patient's unique requirements, symptoms, and preferences, increasing the efficacy of treatment.

- **Real-Time Intervention Alerts:** AI-driven mental health applications can notify physicians and patients when symptoms increase or early warning indicators of a relapse emerge, allowing for prompt support and intervention.

- **Enhanced Patient Outcomes:** AI-driven care can help people manage illnesses with fewer problems by detecting early signs and tracking treatment responses.

6.3 AI in the Identification of Infectious Diseases

AI's quick diagnostic tools, real-time monitoring, and worldwide tracking capabilities have revolutionized the management of infectious diseases. Healthcare systems can efficiently respond to pandemics and other public health emergencies because of these technologies, which are particularly useful in outbreak management and monitoring.

Machine Learning for Viral and Bacterial Infection Detection: AI-powered technologies examine clinical data and patient samples to accurately identify bacterial and viral illnesses, frequently in a fraction of the time needed by conventional techniques.

- **Quick Diagnostic Tests:** Within minutes, machine learning algorithms analyze data from patient samples, including blood or saliva, to detect infections. In urgent care settings, where prompt diagnosis is essential, these tests are particularly helpful.

- **Genomic Sequencing for Pathogen Identification**: Artificial Intelligence (AI) speeds up the genomic sequencing process, allowing real-time identification of certain bacterial or viral strains. This is crucial for differentiating between various infectious agents and customizing treatment plans.

- The ability of AI to detect pathogens at extremely low concentrations has improved diagnostic test sensitivity and specificity, which is crucial for precise identification of infectious diseases, particularly newly developing pathogens.

- **Real-Time Monitoring and Tracking of Infectious**

Diseases: Public health officials may effectively allocate resources and carry out containment measures by monitoring infectious disease outbreaks as they happen thanks to real-time data analysis.

- In order to identify trends and anticipate possible epidemics, artificial intelligence (AI) systems examine data from a variety of sources, including social media, hospital admissions, and even environmental samples.

- **Contact Tracing and Predictive Modeling:** AI-driven applications make it easier to track down contacts by identifying those who have been exposed to infectious diseases, and predictive models forecast the spread of illnesses, assisting public health organizations in taking prompt action.

- **Data-Driven Decision-Making**: AI gives policymakers useful insights to help them make well-informed decisions on vaccination programs, resource distribution, and quarantines by combining data from many sources.

Beyond diagnosis, artificial intelligence (AI) aids in the worldwide management of infectious illnesses by assisting with disease surveillance, outbreak forecasting, and immunization programs.

- **Disease Surveillance Systems:** AI-powered platforms track global data, identifying trends in real time to forecast the probability of infectious disease outbreaks and facilitate prompt action.

- **Vaccination and Treatment Development:** By examining molecular data to find possible therapeutic targets for infectious diseases, AI speeds up the discovery of new drugs and vaccines. AI algorithms aided in the rapid identification of vaccine candidates during the COVID-19 pandemic.

- **Global Health Initiatives:** The World Health Organization (WHO) and other organizations track infectious diseases and coordinate responses across nations using AI-driven data analytics.

There is enormous promise for early diagnosis, better patient outcomes, and more effective illness management using AI applications in infectious, neurological, cardiovascular, and mental health disease detection. AI offers strong capabilities that shorten diagnosis times, improve therapy tailoring, and provide real-time insights into public health trends and illness development by utilizing sophisticated data analysis. Precision medicine will eventually become the norm for the identification and treatment of non-cancer diseases, radically altering how we approach and address pervasive health issues. This is made possible by the ongoing integration of AI into healthcare.

CHAPTER 7

Early Detection and Genetic Testing

A new era of customized medicine has been brought about by genetic testing, which enables the early detection and prevention of a variety of diseases based on a person's genetic composition. Genetic research advancements have made it possible to identify particular markers linked to heightened vulnerability to particular diseases, which has resulted in more specialized diagnostics, preventative actions, and, in certain situations, individualized treatment plans. The importance of genetic markers in illness susceptibility, the cutting-edge diagnostic uses of CRISPR technology, and the privacy and ethical concerns surrounding genetic testing are all covered in this chapter.

7.1 Genetic Indicators of Disease Propensity

With its ability to provide information on a person's risk of developing disorders based on their distinct genetic profile, genetic testing has emerged as a crucial tool in the early detection of diseases. Healthcare professionals can anticipate illness vulnerability, customize preventative measures, and occasionally take action before symptoms appear by detecting particular genetic markers.

Introduction to Genetic Testing in Diagnostics: Genetic testing is the process of examining DNA to find alterations, or mutations, that could cause illness. Genetic testing enables the identification of predispositions long before symptoms manifest, whereas traditional diagnosis relies on observable symptoms and family medical histories. Genetic testing is becoming more affordable and available to a wider range of people because of developments in DNA sequencing technologies.

- **Types of Genetic Testing:** These include pharmacogenomic testing, which predicts a person's reaction to specific drugs; carrier testing, which evaluates the risk of passing a genetic mutation to children; and predictive testing, which calculates the probability of developing a genetic disorder.

- **Clinical Practice Applications:** Genetic testing is frequently used in cardiology, neurology, and oncology, where early identification of risk factors can direct preventative actions. Patients who are at high risk for cardiovascular disease, for instance, can benefit from intensive lifestyle factor management, while those who are at risk for particular cancers might benefit from routine testing.

- In order to assist people understand their risks and make well-informed decisions about preventive or therapeutic actions, genetic counseling is frequently provided in conjunction with genetic testing.

Common Genetic Markers for Cancers and Chronic Illnesses: Certain genetic markers, or gene variations, are linked to a higher chance of developing certain diseases, particularly chronic ailments and cancers.

- **Oncology:** While mutations in genes like TP53 and PTEN are associated with different cancer types, the BRCA1 and BRCA2 gene mutations are well-known indicators of breast and ovarian cancer risk. Proactive observation and potentially life-saving prophylactic interventions can result from the identification of these mutations.
- **Cardiovascular Disease:** High cholesterol and a

higher risk of heart disease are linked to genetic markers like those found in the PCSK9 and LDLR genes. Through genetic testing for these markers, people can minimize risk early on by changing their lifestyle or taking medicine.

- **Diabetes and Autoimmune Disorders:** A higher risk of developing type 2 diabetes and autoimmune illnesses is associated with specific genetic variants, such as those in the HLA and TCF7L2 genes. Changes in food, exercise, and lifestyle can help reduce risk if these signs are found early.

How Genetics Can Indicate Illness Predisposition: Certain genetic variants indicate higher risk factors, and genetics plays a crucial part in illness predisposition. Although genes by themselves do not cause disease, they do increase a person's vulnerability.

- The interplay of genes with environmental variables, lifestyle, and other biological aspects is highlighted by the fact that some people may carry genetic variants that raise their risk yet may never acquire the disease.
- The polygenic risk scores (PRS), which combine the

impacts of several genetic markers to evaluate an individual's risk for complicated diseases like coronary artery disease and type 2 diabetes, are a result of recent advances in genetics. Even if a person does not have high-impact mutations, PRS can still be used to identify high-risk individuals.

7.2 Diagnostic Uses of CRISPR Technology

A potent tool for precision diagnostics, CRISPR (Clustered Regularly Interspaced Short Palindromic Repeats) has become a ground-breaking genome editing method. CRISPR was first created for gene editing, but its uses in diagnostics are growing and enable early disease identification, particularly for viral and genetic disorders.

Basics of CRISPR in Genetic Editing: With previously unheard-of precision, scientists can target and alter particular DNA segments thanks to CRISPR technology. Fundamentally, CRISPR locates the desired DNA sequence using a guide RNA. The Cas9 protein then cuts the DNA like molecular scissors, enabling the insertion, deletion, or modification of genetic material.

- The way CRISPR works is by a lock-and-key system. The Cas9 enzyme is guided to precisely cut at the desired location by the guide RNA, which is made to match a certain DNA sequence.

- **Research Applications:** Beyond diagnostics, CRISPR has transformed gene therapy and research, allowing researchers to examine the consequences of gene mutations and create possible treatments for hereditary illnesses.

CRISPR as a Gene-Related Disease Diagnostic Tool: CRISPR's diagnostic uses include locating certain genetic sequences linked to illnesses, offering quick, precise, and economical diagnoses.

- **SHERLOCK and DETECTR Systems:** By focusing on RNA or DNA sequences linked to disease, these CRISPR-based diagnostic tools can detect pathogens and genetic alterations. For instance, DETECTR has demonstrated potential in detecting cancer mutations, whereas SHERLOCK was created to identify viral RNA sequences and detect infections such as dengue and Zika.

- Point-of-Care Testing: CRISPR-based diagnostics

have the potential to be used for point-of-care testing, which would enable quick illness identification outside of conventional laboratory settings. In places with limited resources, where access to healthcare is restricted, this is especially advantageous.

- **Precision Diagnostics:** CRISPR's specificity guarantees that just the desired genetic sequence is detected, reducing the possibility of false positives and boosting the accuracy of test results.

Potential for tailored Treatment and Early Intervention: By determining unique genetic profiles and adjusting interventions appropriately, CRISPR-based diagnostics can result in tailored treatments.

- **Genotype-Targeted Therapy:** Based on each patient's distinct genetic composition, CRISPR diagnostics can detect mutations in genes such as EGFR in cancer patients, enabling targeted treatments that have a higher chance of success.
- **preventative Healthcare**: CRISPR diagnostics facilitate proactive healthcare by detecting genetic risk factors early. This enables people to lower their

risk of disease by managing lifestyle factors or undergoing preventative procedures.

- **CRISPR Diagnostics' Future:** Scientists are trying to broaden the diagnostic uses of CRISPR to encompass more illnesses and genetic conditions, which will eventually provide access to individualized and preventive care.

7.3 Privacy and Ethical Concerns with Genetic Testing

Genetic testing presents serious ethical and privacy issues even if it has many advantages for individualized care and early disease detection. As genetic testing becomes more common, it is crucial to think about how to handle genetic data, the consequences for healthcare policies, and how to strike a balance between patient rights and innovation.

Privacy problems with Genetic Data: Because genetic information is private and specific to each person, there are privacy problems around its storage, accessibility, and dissemination.

- **Data Security**: If genetic data is not adequately protected, it might be misused and result in identity theft and privacy violations. To protect patient privacy, strong encryption and safe data storage are essential.

- **Genetic Discrimination:** People may experience prejudice from insurers or employers due to a genetic predisposition, which could impact their ability to find employment or obtain reasonably priced health insurance.

- **Informed approval:** Patients, especially when it comes to research or sharing data with third parties, must be fully aware of the implications of genetic testing and provide their approval to the use of their data.

The Impact of Genetic Testing on Healthcare Policies: As genetic testing is incorporated into healthcare more and more, it puts existing regulations pertaining to insurance, privacy, and care access under pressure.

- **Implications for Insurance:** If insurers get access to genetic data, they may use it to modify rates or refuse coverage depending on a patient's genetic risk factors, which might lead to inequities in healthcare access.

- **Regulatory Standards:** To guarantee moral behavior and safeguard patient rights, governments and medical associations are attempting to create standards and regulations for genetic testing. For instance, genetic discrimination in employment and health insurance is illegal in the US under the Genetic Information Nondiscrimination Act (GINA).

- Public health experts can address specific disease risks in communities by using genetic testing to uncover population-level health patterns. It is still difficult to strike a balance between the demands of public health and personal privacy.

Balancing Innovation and Patient Rights: As genetic testing develops, ethical healthcare practice depends on striking a balance between individual rights protection and technical innovation.

- Transparency in Data Use: Organizations that provide genetic testing must be open and honest about how their data will be used, including whether it will be shared with outside parties or utilized for research.

- Patients should maintain control over their genetic

data, including the ability to refuse its usage for commercial or scientific purposes. This is known as "autonomy and patient choice."

- **Ethical Oversight:** In order to ensure that the advantages of genetic testing research initiatives are balanced against any possible harms to participants, ethical review boards are essential.

Early detection technology and genetic testing are a major step forward in personalized healthcare, with the potential to detect and treat illnesses before they manifest. CRISPR technology promises quick and precise tests, while genetic markers offer important insights on disease vulnerability. But as these technologies advance, it will be crucial to address privacy, ethical, and policy issues to guarantee that genetic testing is both morally sound and accessible, protecting patient rights in the precision medicine era.

CHAPTER 8

EARLY DISEASE DETECTION USING WEARABLE TECHNOLOGY

Real-time health monitoring, made possible by wearable technology, has transformed healthcare by promoting early disease identification, preventive care, and better patient outcomes. Wearable technology, ranging from smartwatches and fitness trackers to sophisticated biosensors, continuously gathers health data and offers insightful information that helps detect early symptoms of a number of illnesses. This chapter examines the ways in which wearable technology tracks health indicators, its potential for early disease detection, and the advances and problems influencing wearables' use in healthcare going forward.

8.1 How Wearable Technology Tracks Health Indicators

In recent years, wearable technology has developed

quickly, moving from basic activity trackers to complex gadgets that can track a variety of physiological and biochemical markers. These measures assist users in monitoring their level of fitness and identifying health problems, frequently before symptoms manifest.

Types of Health Metrics Measured by Wearables: These days, wearables measure a variety of health metrics that provide information about an individual's health and possible hazards. Among these metrics are:

1. **Heart Rate:** Wearables monitor resting heart rate, heart rate variability, and even changes during physical exercise, making it a key indicator of cardiovascular health. An underlying cardiovascular problem may be indicated by a heart rate that is consistently elevated or erratic.

2. **Blood Oxygen Saturation (SpO2):** Oxygen saturation measurements can identify respiratory illnesses, sleep apnea, and COVID-19 in addition to revealing respiratory efficiency. SpO2 sensors, which continually detect oxygen levels, are found in many contemporary wearables.

3. **Electrocardiogram (ECG):** Single-lead ECGs,

which identify irregular cardiac rhythms such atrial fibrillation, can be performed by certain wearables. This information aids in the early detection of arrhythmias that, if left untreated, may result in stroke.

4. **Blood Pressure:** Cutting-edge wearable technology uses blood pressure monitoring to reveal information on hypertensive tendencies, which raise the risk of stroke and heart disease.

5. Wearable technology monitors physical activity, sleep quality, and steps taken. Physical activity levels aid in tracking fitness and metabolic health, whereas sleep patterns, in particular, can reveal mental health problems or chronic disorders.

6. **Respiratory Rate:** Wearables can give early signals about infection or respiratory distress by monitoring breaths per minute.

7. **Blood Glucose Levels:** Non-invasive glucose monitoring is becoming a feature of emerging wearable technology. This is revolutionary for people with diabetes because it enables continuous tracking without the need for finger pricks.

The following are some advantages of using wearables to continuously monitor health parameters for the purpose of preventing disease:

- **Early Detection:** Tracking changes in health measurements over time aids in identifying anomalies that may point to the onset of disease. For example, a slight but steady increase in resting heart rate may indicate stress or an approaching disease.

- **Proactive Health Management**: Based on real-time data, individuals are empowered to make informed lifestyle choices, such as bettering their food, exercise, or sleeping patterns, by receiving ongoing feedback on their health state.

- **Reducing Healthcare Burden:** By identifying health problems early, wearables can help ease the burden on healthcare systems by reducing ER visits and enabling prompt interventions.

Wearables in Cardiovascular Health Management: Since heart disease is still one of the world's top causes of death, wearables have mostly focused on cardiovascular health. Wearable technology greatly aids in the early detection and treatment of heart disease by monitoring cardiovascular parameters.

- **Heart Rate and Arrhythmias:** By detecting abnormal heartbeats, devices such as the Apple Watch can notify users of potential arrhythmias, such as atrial fibrillation, that might otherwise go undetected until a serious incident happens.

- **Blood Pressure and Heart Failure**: For people who are at risk of hypertension or heart failure, wearables that measure blood pressure offer useful information. Healthcare professionals can modify medication or lifestyle recommendations for patients with chronic diseases based on real-time data thanks to continuous monitoring.

- **Cholesterol and Lifestyle Tracking**: Although wearables cannot measure cholesterol directly, lifestyle factors such as sleep patterns and activity levels are linked to cardiovascular health, which makes them useful for patients trying to lower their blood pressure or cholesterol through lifestyle changes.

8.2 Early Disease Detection using Wearables

The uses of wearable technology are growing beyond cardiovascular monitoring and fitness tracking. Wearable technology of today is essential for spotting early indicators of metabolic, cardiovascular, and respiratory diseases and providing useful information that may be able to postpone or prevent the start of disease.

Identifying Respiratory, Cardiovascular, and Metabolic Disorders: Wearable technology with cutting-edge sensors can identify a number of acute and chronic illnesses early on.

- **Respiratory Disorders**: Sleep apnea, respiratory infections, and diseases like COPD can be identified using devices equipped with SpO2 and respiratory rate sensors. Wearables give information about respiratory health and enable early intervention by monitoring changes in respiratory rate and oxygen saturation.

- **Cardiovascular Disorders**: Wearables can evaluate general heart health and identify disorders like hypertension and heart failure risk in addition to identifying arrhythmias. Blood pressure monitors are essential for people with hypertension, and wearables with ECG capabilities can detect atrial fibrillation and other arrhythmias.

- **Metabolic Disorders:** By enabling continuous blood glucose monitoring, wearable glucose monitors are revolutionizing the treatment of diabetes. By offering information about the body's glucose metabolism, these gadgets help people with diabetes control their disease and those who are at risk take preventative measures.

Instances of Wearables with an Early Detection Focus: A range of wearables, each with special features aimed at particular medical requirements, are advancing the field of early illness detection.

- With its SpO2 and ECG monitoring features, the Apple Watch is a popular tool for monitoring heart health and identifying atrial fibrillation.
- **Fitbit:** Although it is primarily a fitness tracker, more recent models have stress management and SpO2 monitoring capabilities that are beneficial for overall wellness and can reveal early signs of disease.
- By monitoring strain, sleep, and heart rate

variability, WHOOP focuses on fitness and recovery. It provides insights that can be helpful in spotting times of high physical or mental stress, which are associated with early indicators of sickness.

- Continuous glucose monitors, such as the FreeStyle Libre and Dexcom G6, provide real-time input to individuals with diabetes and serve as an early warning system for those at risk for the disease.

- **Biostrap**: This wearable device provides sophisticated respiration rate tracking and heart rate variability, which are useful for tracking changes in cardiac and respiratory health as well as for monitoring the quality of sleep and recuperation.

Incorporating Wearable Data with Medical Records: By incorporating wearable data into electronic medical records (EMRs), a more comprehensive picture of a patient's health can be produced, enabling more individualized treatment and well-informed decision-making.

- Healthcare providers can create more successful treatment regimens by using wearable data, which gives them a comprehensive picture of the patient's lifestyle, including activity, sleep, and stress levels.

- **Remote Patient Monitoring**: Clinicians can monitor patients with chronic illnesses remotely by integrating wearable data with EMRs. This eliminates the need for frequent hospital visits and enables early intervention in the event that crucial parameters change unexpectedly.

- **Data Standardization:** Wearable data must be interoperable with EMR systems and standardized for successful integration. In order to overcome this difficulty, standards like HL7 FHIR are being developed, which enable wearable data to be easily shared across various healthcare platforms.

8.3 Wearable Technology: Innovations and Challenges

Even with wearable technology's advantages in healthcare, there are still a number of obstacles to overcome. To improve the efficacy of wearables, developers and healthcare providers must solve a number of crucial difficulties, including data accuracy, privacy concerns, integration challenges, and the requirement for sophisticated sensor technologies.

Data Accuracy and Integration Issues: For wearables to be useful in healthcare, they must generate accurate and dependable data. But some restrictions still exist.

- **Sensor Limitations**: Skin tone, user movement, and device positioning are some of the variables that can affect how accurate wearable sensors are. To guarantee accurate health measures, sensor accuracy must be increased.

- Data incompatibility and a lack of standardization are the major reasons why many healthcare organizations find it difficult to integrate wearable data with current EMRs. In order to solve this, developers are developing interoperable systems that smoothly integrate wearable data.

- **User Compliance:** Wearables rely on users to wear and care for the gadget on a regular basis. Maintaining wearability, comfort, and user involvement is essential for accurate data and long-term monitoring.

Innovations in Sensor Technology and Data Analytics: Some of the drawbacks of wearable health monitoring are being addressed by technological developments in sensors and data analytics.

- **Advanced Biosensors:** These new biosensors are able to identify a wider variety of health indicators, including blood glucose, hydration levels, and even mental health biomarkers. Better disease monitoring and prediction are made possible by the development of more precise and sensitive sensors.

- **Machine Learning Algorithms:** Wearable data analysis heavily relies on AI and machine learning. These algorithms help transform raw data into actionable insights by processing vast amounts of data to find tiny patterns and correlations that can forecast the start of illness.

- **Miniaturization and Design:** Wearables are now more comfortable and adaptable thanks to advancements in miniaturization and design. Users find it easier to incorporate wearables into their daily life as compliance and usability improve and devices become less intrusive.

Privacy Issues and Data Security in Wearable Technology: Because health data is sensitive, privacy and security are major issues in wearable technology.

- **Access Control and Data Encryption:** Protecting users requires making sure wearable data is encrypted and that only authorized parties may access it.

Privacy.

- **Regulatory Compliance:** To protect patient data and guarantee the ethical treatment of personal information, healthcare organizations and wearable manufacturers must abide by laws such as HIPAA in the United States and GDPR in Europe.

- **User Awareness and Control**: Wearable technology can be more widely accepted and used if users are given more control over what information is shared and are educated about data privacy.

Significant advancements in early disease identification and health monitoring are still being made by wearable technologies. Wearables give people and healthcare professionals valuable data that can result in earlier interventions and improved health outcomes by measuring important health variables in real-time. However, stakeholders must address current issues with accuracy, integration, and data protection while driving advancements in sensor technology and analytics if wearable technology is to reach its full potential. Wearable technology is expected to play a key role in customized medicine and preventive healthcare as the field develops.

CHAPTER 9

Diagnostics Using Advanced Imaging Technologies

Advanced imaging technologies are essential to diagnostics in the ever changing field of medicine because they allow medical professionals to see the fine intricacies of the human body and identify disorders earlier than ever before. The importance of molecular imaging for early illness detection, the most recent advancements in medical imaging technology, and the advancements in real-time imaging that are revolutionizing surgical techniques and diagnostic precision are all covered in this chapter.

9.1 Advances in Imaging Technologies for Medicine

The ability to identify and track a variety of medical disorders has been greatly improved by recent developments in medical imaging. Significant advancements in resolution and speed have been made in methods like Positron Emission Tomography (PET),

Computed Tomography (CT), and Magnetic Resonance Imaging (MRI), enabling more efficient early disease diagnosis.

The latest developments in MRI, CT, and PET scans for early detection are as follows:

- Over the past ten years, medical imaging has advanced significantly, especially in the areas of MRI, CT, and PET technologies.

- Higher field strengths, such as 3 Tesla (3T) and beyond, have been made possible by advancements in MRI technology, which enhance contrast and picture resolution. By identifying variations in blood flow, innovations such as functional magnetic resonance imaging (fMRI) allow for the viewing of brain activity and can aid in the early detection of neurological diseases.

- **CT:** Multi-detector CT (MDCT) scanners provide quick image capture, which reduces radiation exposure and produces better images. Image reconstruction is improved by sophisticated algorithms, which helps find tiny tumors or lesions that earlier imaging techniques could have overlooked. Lung cancer screening now frequently involves CT scans, which help identify potentially deadly diseases early.

- **PET**: In oncology, PET scans are being utilized more and more to detect cancer early. Recent developments in radiotracers, which are chemicals that show metabolic activity, have increased the sensitivity and specificity of these scans, making it possible to find cancers that traditional imaging methods cannot see.

How Imaging Innovations Enhance Diagnostic Accuracy: Effective patient management and treatment choices depend on the precision of diagnostic imaging. Advances in imaging technologies have increased the precision of diagnosis by:

- **Higher Resolution Images:** Improved imaging methods yield sharper, more detailed images, which enable radiologists and physicians to interpret them more precisely.
- **Artificial Intelligence (AI) Integration:** To help with picture interpretation, AI algorithms are being included into imaging workflows more and more.

Early and more precise diagnoses can result from the use of machine learning algorithms to spot patterns and abnormalities in photos that the human eye would miss.

- **Multimodal Imaging:** By offering complementary information about the structure and metabolism of tissues, combining various imaging modalities (such as PET/CT or PET/MRI) improves diagnostic accuracy. A more thorough evaluation of illnesses is made possible by this integrative method, especially in cancer.

Image-Guided Biopsies for Specific Cancers: Image-guided biopsy methods, such CT, MRI, or ultrasound-guided biopsies, have completely changed the way biopsies are carried out, especially when it comes to cancer diagnosis.

- **Precision Targeting:** By precisely aiming tumors, these methods reduce the possibility of problems and boost the production of tissue samples for diagnostic purposes. For example, CT-guided biopsies can be used to collect samples from nodules that are otherwise challenging to reach in lung cancer cases.

- **Minimally Invasive:** Compared to standard surgical biopsies, image-guided biopsies are usually less invasive, which shortens recovery times and lessens patient suffering.

- The capacity to see the tumor during the biopsy process greatly increases the likelihood of collecting a sufficient sample for pathological investigation, which is essential for precise diagnosis and treatment planning. This results in a Enhanced Diagnostic Yield.

9.2 Molecular Imaging to Identify Diseases Early

A revolutionary method in diagnostics, molecular imaging makes it possible to see biological processes at the molecular and cellular levels. For the early detection of diseases, this technology is very helpful in cardiology, neurology, and oncology.

Molecular Imaging's Role in Disease diagnosis: By using particular biomarkers, molecular imaging techniques offer insights into cellular processes and activities, enabling the early diagnosis of diseases.

- **Biomarkers and Radiotracers:** These imaging methods frequently use radiotracers, which attach to particular cellular targets and provide details on the molecular composition of tissues. For instance, the radiotracer fluorodeoxyglucose (FDG) is frequently used in PET scans to identify regions with elevated glucose metabolism, which is frequently a sign of tumor activity.

- **Non-Invasive Assessment:** Since molecular imaging is non-invasive, it offers a special chance to track the course of a disease and its response to treatment without requiring surgery.

One of the most important benefits of molecular imaging is its capacity to detect early pathological changes before structural abnormalities become noticeable. This is known as "Detecting Early Cancerous Changes at the Cellular Level."

- **Cellular and Molecular Changes:** Cancers can be identified in their early stages thanks to molecular imaging, which can identify metabolic changes linked to tumor growth. This capacity is essential for tumors since better patient outcomes depend on early intervention.

- The insights obtained from molecular imaging can help with individualized treatment approaches by detecting particular tumor traits. This allows for targeted medicines that increase efficacy while reducing negative effects.

Impact on Treatment Outcomes and Survival Rates: Treatment outcomes and survival rates are greatly impacted by the capacity to identify diseases early.

- **Timely therapies:** Molecular imaging enables early diagnosis, allowing for prompt therapies that can improve prognosis for patients with diseases like cancer. According to research, individuals who receive an early diagnosis have a much higher chance of surviving.

- **Monitoring therapy Response:** Molecular imaging is also essential for tracking therapy response, which allows physicians to modify treatments in real time depending on feedback about how well they are working.

9.3 Real-Time Imaging in Diagnosis and Surgery

The way treatments are carried out and diagnoses are made has been completely transformed by the incorporation of real-time imaging technologies into surgical and diagnostic techniques. These developments improve patient outcomes, decrease invasiveness, and increase precision.

Advances in Real-Time Imaging During Surgeries: MRI, fluoroscopy, and intraoperative ultrasonography are examples of real-time imaging technologies that give surgeons instant visual input while doing surgeries.

- **Guided Surgery:** Surgeons may precisely navigate intricate anatomical structures with real-time imaging, reducing injury to surrounding tissues. To ensure total resection while maintaining vital brain processes, neurosurgeons can use intraoperative magnetic resonance imaging (MRI) to see brain tumors in real time.

- **Immediate Decision Making:** Having access to real-time imaging during surgery enables prompt decision-making, allowing for modifications based on existing circumstances and improving overall surgical results.

Improving Accuracy and Reducing Invasive operations: Real-time structural visualization improves accuracy during minimally invasive operations.

- **Decreased Complications:** Real-time imaging speeds up recovery and lessens postoperative discomfort by allowing surgeons to precisely target particular locations, lowering the likelihood of complications related to open surgery.

- **Expanded Surgical Possibilities:** Real-time imaging technologies increase the range of what may be achieved with minimally invasive techniques by making it possible to execute complex procedures that may have previously needed invasive approaches.

Future of Real-Time Imaging in Early Diagnosis: As imaging technology advances, real-time imaging has a bright future ahead of it in terms of early diagnosis.

- **Integration of AI and Machine Learning:** By integrating AI algorithms with real-time imaging, anomalies can be automatically detected during imaging operations, potentially improving diagnostic capabilities.

- **Advances in Imaging Modalities:** New imaging modalities, such optical coherence tomography and photoacoustic imaging, are being developed to provide real-time feedback at previously unheard-of resolutions, which could enable early cellular disease identification.

- **Telemedicine Applications:** By combining real-time imaging with telemedicine platforms, specialists might conduct remote surgical consultations, improving access to sophisticated treatment, particularly in underprivileged areas, and allowing them to direct procedures from a distance.

Modern medicine's diagnostic and therapeutic landscape is changing as a result of advanced imaging technology. While molecular imaging tools offer insights into disease processes at the cellular level, advancements in MRI, CT, and PET scans improve early illness diagnosis. New developments in real-time imaging are transforming surgery, improving patient outcomes and precision. In order to improve patient care and survival rates, early diagnosis and efficient disease management will become more and more dependent on the incorporation of these technologies into clinical practice as they develop.

CHAPTER 10

TECHNOLOGY'S ROLE IN EARLY DETECTION AND DISEASE PREVENTION

The application of cutting-edge technologies to early diagnosis and illness prevention has the potential to significantly alter patient care as the healthcare industry develops. The future of technology in this crucial field is examined in this chapter, with particular attention paid to predictive analytics in preventive healthcare, upcoming prospects and difficulties, and new developments in early disease detection technologies.

10.1 Preventive healthcare and predictive analytics

Predictive analytics, which uses data and statistical algorithms to determine the likelihood of future outcomes based on prior data, is quickly becoming a key component of preventative healthcare. This strategy gives medical professionals the ability to act sooner, maybe preventing the beginning of illnesses before they worsen.

Predictive Models in Preventive Medicine: To predict health risks, predictive models use massive datasets such as genomic data, lifestyle data, and electronic health records (EHRs).

- **Risk Stratification:** Predictive algorithms can categorize patients according to their likelihood of contracting particular diseases, such diabetes or heart disease, by examining patterns and trends within patient populations. By allowing for customized therapies targeted at high-risk people, this classification greatly improves preventive care.

- **Machine Learning Algorithms:** To improve prediction models, sophisticated machine learning methods are being used more and more. The accuracy of risk forecasts can be increased by using these algorithms to find intricate linkages in the data that conventional statistical techniques might miss.

Proactive Monitoring and Risk Assessments: Improving patient outcomes requires a change in healthcare from reactive to proactive.

- **Continuous Monitoring:** Health parameters like blood pressure, heart rate, and activity levels may be continuously monitored thanks to wearable technology and mobile health apps. Healthcare professionals can spot early warning indicators of possible health problems and take action before they worsen thanks to this real-time data collecting.

- A patient's health can be seen holistically by implementing comprehensive risk assessments that take lifestyle, environmental, and hereditary factors into account. By encouraging better habits and lowering the risk of disease development, these evaluations can help guide individualized preventative plans.

Benefits for Patient Outcomes and Healthcare Costs: Predictive analytics integration in preventative healthcare offers significant financial advantages in addition to improving patient outcomes.

- **Improved Health Outcomes:** Better chronic disease management can result from early detection and intervention, which lowers the risk of complications and hospital stays. For instance, those who have been determined to be at high risk for heart disease may benefit from lifestyle modifications and prescription drugs to effectively control their risk factors.

- **Cost Savings**: Healthcare systems can drastically cut treatment and hospitalization expenses by preventing the start of diseases. By lowering healthcare costs, investments in predictive analytics and preventative healthcare can yield a sizable return on investment.

10.2 Healthcare Technology: Opportunities and Challenges

Although technology holds great promise for illness prevention and early diagnosis, a number of obstacles must be overcome before its full potential can be realized. There are a lot of chances for innovation and better healthcare delivery when these issues are acknowledged and resolved.

Regulatory and Ethical Challenges: In order to protect patient safety and data privacy, significant ethical and regulatory issues are brought up by the adoption of new technologies in the healthcare industry.

- **Regulatory Oversight**: In order to properly assess and authorize new technology, regulatory authorities need to create frameworks. The adoption of advantageous technologies is frequently delayed because the speed at which technology is developing frequently surpasses the capabilities of current regulatory procedures.

- **Ethical Implications**: Informed permission, data ownership, and potential biases in algorithmic decision-making are among the ethical issues brought up by the application of predictive analytics and data-driven methodologies. Building public trust requires making sure that these technologies are used in an ethical and responsible manner.

Integrating Emerging Tech into Healthcare Systems: Stakeholder participation and meticulous planning are necessary for the effective integration of emerging technologies into current healthcare systems.

- **Interoperability:** Interoperability across many platforms and systems is essential to the effectiveness of predictive analytics and other technologies. To enable smooth data interchange between healthcare institutions, standardization of data formats and communication protocols is necessary.

- **Education and Training:** In order to use new technology in their practice, healthcare providers need to be properly trained. This involves being able to decipher predictive analytics and apply them to clinical judgment.

Crossing the Gap Between Tech Advancements and Healthcare acceptance: Although technology has a lot of potential, it can be difficult to close the gap between innovation and real-world acceptance in the healthcare industry.

- Involving patients, legislators, and healthcare professionals in the creation and application of new technologies is essential for promoting adoption and guaranteeing that these solutions satisfy end users' expectations.

- **Demonstrating Value:** By proving the concrete advantages of new technologies through evidence-based research and pilot programs, stakeholders can be convinced of their worth, which will encourage broader adoption and integration into standard practice.

10.3 Upcoming Developments in Technologies for Early Disease Identification

Thanks to developments in wearable technology, nanotechnology, and artificial intelligence, early disease detection is set to undergo revolutionary changes in the future. By improving the capacity to detect illnesses in their early stages, these trends are reshaping the healthcare industry.

Growth Areas in Diagnostics and Treatment: Early disease identification through a variety of cutting-edge techniques is the main focus of the rapidly growing field of diagnostics.

- **Liquid Biopsy:** By analyzing circulating tumor cells and cell-free DNA in the blood, liquid biopsies are becoming a non-invasive way to find cancer. This method eliminates the need for invasive tissue biopsies and enables early tumor diagnosis and surveillance.

- Diagnostic tests can now be conducted at the patient's bedside or in public places because of advancements in point-of-care testing. Especially in emergency and primary care settings, these quick tests facilitate prompt decision-making and early interventions.

Future-Shaping Role of AI, Nanotech, and Wearables: The combination of advanced technologies like wearables, nanotechnology, and artificial intelligence is revolutionizing early disease diagnosis.

- The use of artificial intelligence (AI) algorithms to evaluate large volumes of health data is growing, which enhances diagnostic precision and makes early disease detection possible. Faster and more precise diagnosis is made possible by machine learning models' ability to spot patterns and abnormalities in imaging, genomic, and clinical data.
- **Nanotechnology:** By creating nanosensors that can identify biomolecules at extremely low concentrations, nanotechnology provides innovative methods for disease detection. Early disease detection from these sensors may allow for treatment

to begin before symptoms appear.

- **Wearable Devices:** Vital signs and health measurements may be continuously monitored thanks to the widespread use of wearable technology, such as smartwatches and health trackers. As these gadgets advance, they will be able to deliver real-time information that warns patients and medical professionals of possible health problems.

Prospects for Widespread Adoption of Early Detection Tech: As technology advances, there seems to be a good chance that early detection technologies will be widely used in the medical field.

- **Increased Patient Involvement:** As consumer health technology proliferates, consumers are being empowered to actively participate in their own health care. Preventive healthcare practices and the need for early detection solutions may be fueled by this shift toward patient engagement.

- **Integration into Standard Practice:** Healthcare systems are likely to incorporate early detection technologies into standard clinical practice as proof of their efficacy grows. To guarantee that innovations satisfy clinical demands and are in line with patient care goals, this integration will necessitate constant cooperation between technology developers, healthcare providers, and legislators.

There is enormous promise for the use of technology in early disease identification and prevention in the future. Proactive monitoring and predictive analytics have intriguing opportunities to enhance patient outcomes and lower healthcare expenses. There are still many obstacles to overcome, including ethical and legal issues, but there are also a lot of chances for creativity. The potential for broad adoption of early detection technologies will continue to transform the healthcare landscape as we embrace new diagnostic trends like artificial intelligence (AI), nanotechnology, and wearable technology. This will encourage a more proactive approach to illness prevention and health management.

ABOUT THE AUTHOR

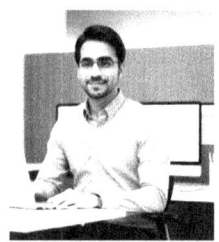 Technology specialist and author Emma Royce Smartley specializes in the newest developments in AI, coding tools, and software development. His goal as a writer is to help developers and tech fans remain ahead of the curve by simplifying difficult tech ideas. His publications provide insightful analyses of how new technologies are changing the landscape of productivity and software development. Emma's love of innovation propels him to investigate and elucidate the technologies that will shape the landscape of the future.

www.ingramcontent.com/pod-product-compliance
Lightning Source LLC
Chambersburg PA
CBHW071518220526
45472CB00003B/1071